Historical Breakouts of the Mpox

From 1958 to 2024

Ashley Green

5

Table of Contents

Introduction: The History of Monkeypox Outbreaks

The year is 1958. In a remote research facility in Copenhagen, Denmark, a group of scientists are studying a colony of monkeys. The goal: to understand the mysterious disease that is ravaging the primates, a disease marked by fever, rashes, and lesions. The scientists are unaware that their work will soon become a crucial piece of a global puzzle, a puzzle that stretches across decades, continents, and lives. This is the story of monkeypox, a virus that emerged from the depths of the African rainforest and has, over the last 70 years, captivated and terrified the world.

While the story of monkeypox is rooted in the discovery of the virus in those Copenhagen monkeys, its origins lie far deeper, nestled within the intricate web of life in Central and West Africa. The virus, a member of the Orthopoxvirus genus, shares a lineage with smallpox, a disease that ravaged humanity for centuries. But unlike smallpox, monkeypox had long remained hidden, a silent threat lurking within the diverse ecosystem of the African tropics.

This book delves into the history of monkeypox, chronicling its evolution from an obscure viral threat confined to the dense jungles of Africa to a global concern. We will explore the early discoveries, the first outbreaks, and the gradual emergence of the virus onto the world stage. We will trace its journey from a disease primarily affecting monkeys and rodents to one capable of crossing the species barrier and infecting humans, leading to a series of outbreaks that have left their mark on medical history.

The narrative unfolds in six distinct chapters, each serving as a window into a crucial period of monkeypox's evolution:

Chapter 1: Initial Discovery (1950s-1970s): This chapter takes us to the heart of the discovery, delving into the research that brought monkeypox to the attention of scientists. We explore the early understanding of the virus, its initial characterization, and the realization that it posed a potential threat to human health. We will examine the role of animal research, the identification of the virus's natural reservoir, and the initial attempts to control its spread.

Chapter 2: Early Outbreaks (1980s-1990s): Here, we transition from the scientific realm to the human one, chronicling the emergence of the first human monkeypox outbreaks. These early outbreaks, confined largely to Central and West Africa, were largely confined to rural communities and primarily affected children. We will examine the unique characteristics of these outbreaks, the public health responses, and the growing concern about the virus's potential for spread.

Chapter 3: Emergence in the United States (2003): This chapter marks a pivotal moment in the history of monkeypox. It recounts the first outbreak of the virus on American soil, a series of cases linked to the importation of pet prairie dogs from Ghana. This event not only highlighted the potential for international travel and trade to facilitate the spread of monkeypox but also triggered a major public health response and a renewed focus on the virus's potential impact on the global community.

Chapter 4: Continued Activity in Africa (2000s-2010s): While the United States outbreak in 2003 sent shockwaves through the world, monkeypox continued to circulate in its endemic region, Africa. This chapter explores the continued presence of the virus in Central and West Africa, analyzing the patterns of outbreaks, the evolving understanding of its epidemiology, and the challenges faced by local health authorities in containing the virus.

Chapter 5: Global Concern and Spread (2020s): The 2020s ushered in a new era of monkeypox. This chapter explores the rapid spread of the virus beyond its traditional endemic regions, a phenomenon linked to increased global travel, trade, and a changing world. We examine the factors that contributed to this surge, analyze the impact of the spread on various countries and regions, and delve into the evolving public health response to this global crisis.

Chapter 6: Ongoing Developments (2023-Present): This chapter delves into the present-day reality of monkeypox, exploring the ongoing efforts to control the spread of the virus, the ongoing research into its epidemiology and treatment options, and the potential for future outbreaks. We will explore the evolving landscape of monkeypox, the challenges that lie ahead, and the ongoing efforts to develop effective prevention and control strategies.

The story of monkeypox is one of scientific discovery, human resilience, and the constant struggle to understand and control infectious diseases. This book is a testament to the remarkable journey of this virus, a journey that highlights the interconnectedness of our world and the critical role of public health in safeguarding human well-being. By delving into the history of monkeypox outbreaks, we gain invaluable insights into the nature of viral evolution, the challenges of pandemic preparedness, and the importance of international collaboration in addressing global health threats.

Chapter 1: Initial Discovery (1950s-1970s)

1.1 A Shadow in the Jungle: The First Encounter

The year is 1958. In the heart of Copenhagen, Denmark, a research facility buzzes with activity. Scientists, driven by a thirst for knowledge and a desire to understand the intricate workings of nature, are studying a colony of monkeys. These primates, native to the jungles of West Africa, have been imported for research purposes, and their health is a primary concern. It is within this setting, amidst the bustling scientific pursuit, that the first encounter with monkeypox, a silent, lurking threat, takes place.

The research team, led by Danish scientist Preben von Magnus, observes a perplexing illness among the monkeys. Fever, lethargy, and characteristic skin lesions - these are the telltale signs of a disease that is both alarming and mysterious. The scientists, meticulously documenting their observations, note the distinctive features of the lesions - small, raised bumps that evolve into pustules, leaving behind scars.

The world has never seen this disease before. The team painstakingly isolates the infectious agent responsible for this ailment, revealing a virus belonging to the Orthopoxvirus genus - a family closely related to the dreaded smallpox virus. This newly identified virus, named *monkeypox*, becomes the first known member of the Orthopoxvirus genus beyond smallpox itself. The discovery of monkeypox marks a pivotal moment in the history of viral diseases, prompting a surge of scientific curiosity and a growing awareness of a potential threat.

1.2 A Glimpse into the Reservoir: The Link to Rodents

The initial discovery of monkeypox in the Copenhagen monkey colony raises crucial questions. Where did this virus originate? What is its natural reservoir, the animal species within which it quietly resides and thrives? The answer to these questions would be crucial in understanding the potential for monkeypox to spill over into human populations.

Intriguingly, the infected monkeys exhibited no signs of the disease upon arrival in Copenhagen. The virus, it seemed, had struck them only after they had been housed together in the research facility. This observation pointed towards a possible route of transmission – a shared environment, perhaps an infected animal or insect, that served as a vector.

Through careful investigation, the scientists trace the source of the outbreak to a shipment of African gray monkeys from Ghana. However, the monkeys themselves were not the original source of the virus. The culprit was identified as a small, furry mammal – a rodent. This discovery is a significant breakthrough, as it reveals the natural reservoir of monkeypox: a group of animals that play an essential role in the virus's life cycle and its potential to spread.

The identification of rodents as the primary reservoir has profound implications. It suggests that monkeypox is a zoonotic disease, meaning it can jump from animals to humans. This discovery underscores the intimate connection between human and animal health, highlighting the importance of understanding the complex interplay between wildlife and human societies.

1.3 The Early Years: Limited Outbreaks and Emerging Concerns

The initial discovery of monkeypox in 1958 marked the beginning of a long journey, a journey of scientific investigation, public health surveillance, and the gradual unfolding of the virus's true nature.

The years following the discovery witnessed the emergence of sporadic outbreaks of monkeypox, primarily in Central and West Africa. The outbreaks were mostly confined to rural communities, primarily affecting children who were in close contact with infected animals, particularly rodents.

These early outbreaks, though limited in scope, provided invaluable insights into the epidemiology of monkeypox. The transmission pattern, characterized by close contact with infected animals or individuals, became evident. The severity of the disease, while generally mild, could cause significant discomfort and, in rare cases, lead to complications like pneumonia or encephalitis.

The early years of research into monkeypox were marked by limited resources and scientific understanding. The virus was still poorly understood, and the lack of effective treatments and vaccines left public health officials with limited tools to address outbreaks. Yet, these early outbreaks served as a crucial wake-up call, sparking a growing concern about the potential for monkeypox to emerge as a global health threat.

1.4 The Emergence of a Potential Pandemic

The 1970s saw a significant shift in the understanding of monkeypox. While outbreaks remained confined to Africa, the scientific community recognized the potential for the virus to spread beyond its endemic region. This concern was fueled by the increasing interconnectedness of the world, driven by globalization and international travel.

The realization that monkeypox could pose a global threat sparked intensified research efforts. Scientists worked tirelessly to understand the virus's genetic makeup, its transmission dynamics, and its potential for adaptation. The race was on to develop effective diagnostic tools, vaccines, and antiviral treatments.

The 1970s marked a pivotal turning point in the history of monkeypox. The virus, once confined to the depths of the African jungle, had begun to cast a long shadow, raising anxieties and prompting urgent calls for global preparedness. The world was on the cusp of a new era, an era defined by the potential for emerging infectious diseases, including monkeypox, to disrupt the delicate balance of human health.

1.5 The Importance of Early Discovery: A Legacy of Learning

The discovery of monkeypox in the 1950s, though seemingly insignificant at the time, proved to be a pivotal moment in the history of public health. The initial encounter with the virus, confined to a research facility in Copenhagen, was a prelude to a story that would unfold across decades, continents, and countless lives.

The early research into monkeypox, fueled by scientific curiosity and a commitment to understanding infectious diseases, laid the groundwork for the future. The identification of the virus's natural reservoir in rodents, the recognition of the potential for human infection, and the early attempts to develop diagnostic tools and vaccines were all crucial steps in preparing the world for the challenges that lay ahead.

The legacy of the initial discovery of monkeypox is a testament to the power of scientific inquiry. It underscores the importance of vigilance, early detection, and a commitment to understanding the intricate relationship between human health and the natural world. As we venture into the following chapters, we will delve deeper into the complex history of monkeypox, tracing its evolution from a remote jungle threat to a global concern. The lessons learned from the early years of discovery will serve as a guide, reminding us of the critical importance of scientific progress and global collaboration in safeguarding human health.

Chapter 2: Early Outbreaks (1980s-1990s)

2.1 A Shadow Emerges: The First Human Outbreaks

The 1980s marked a significant shift in the history of monkeypox. While the virus had been identified in monkeys in the 1950s, it remained largely confined to its natural reservoir, primarily rodents, in the dense rainforests of Central and West Africa. However, the decade saw the emergence of the first documented human outbreaks, a stark reminder of the virus's potential to cross the species barrier and impact human health.

The initial human outbreaks were primarily confined to rural communities in the Democratic Republic of Congo (DRC), formerly Zaire, and other parts of Central Africa. These outbreaks were often characterized by a relatively small number of cases, typically affecting children who were in close contact with infected animals, particularly rodents.

The first human monkeypox outbreak in the DRC, reported in 1981, involved a small number of cases clustered in a remote village. The infected individuals, primarily children, presented with the characteristic symptoms: fever, headache, muscle aches, and a distinctive rash that evolved into pustules. The outbreak, though small, served as a crucial wake-up call, signaling the virus's potential to spill over into human populations and prompting increased public health surveillance efforts.

2.2 Tracing the Source: The Role of Rodents and Wildlife

The emergence of human monkeypox outbreaks raised crucial questions about the transmission dynamics of the virus. Early research focused on identifying the source of infection, the specific animals that served as the link between the virus's natural reservoir and human populations.

Studies conducted in the 1980s and 1990s revealed the crucial role of rodents in the transmission cycle. Rodents, particularly the African giant pouched rat (Cricetomys gambianus), were identified as the primary reservoir of the virus. These rodents were found to carry the virus and shed it in their saliva, urine, and feces, creating a potential pathway for human infection.

The transmission often occurred through direct contact with infected rodents, such as handling them during hunting or farming activities. However, indirect transmission was also possible, through contact with contaminated environments, such as rodent burrows, or through the bite of infected insects.

The outbreaks in the 1980s also highlighted the potential role of other wildlife species in the transmission cycle. While rodents were considered the primary reservoir, other animals, including monkeys, could become infected and potentially transmit the virus to humans. However, the role of these other species in the transmission cycle was less clear and required further investigation.

2.3 A Silent Threat: The Challenges of Diagnosing and Managing Monkeypox

One of the major challenges faced during the early outbreaks was the difficulty in diagnosing monkeypox. The symptoms, while distinctive, could be confused with other viral diseases, including smallpox, chickenpox, and measles. This lack of readily available diagnostic tests often led to delays in diagnosis, making it difficult to track the spread of the virus and implement effective public health measures.

The lack of a specific treatment for monkeypox further complicated the management of outbreaks. The virus, being closely related to smallpox, was susceptible to some antiviral medications used to treat smallpox, but these medications were not readily available or widely used in many African countries. The management of monkeypox outbreaks often relied on supportive care, including symptom management, fluid replacement, and infection control measures.

The challenges of diagnosing and managing monkeypox in the 1980s and 1990s highlighted the urgent need for improved diagnostic tools, effective treatments, and a better understanding of the virus's transmission dynamics. These early outbreaks served as a stark reminder of the potential threat posed by emerging infectious diseases, particularly those with zoonotic origins.

2.4 A Focus on Public Health: Early Interventions and Surveillance

The emergence of human monkeypox outbreaks in the 1980s prompted a renewed focus on public health efforts to prevent and control the spread of the virus. These efforts were largely centered around education, surveillance, and the implementation of infection control measures.

Public health campaigns were launched to educate communities about the risks of monkeypox and the importance of avoiding contact with infected animals. These campaigns emphasized the role of rodents in the transmission cycle and provided guidance on safe handling practices for hunting, farming, and handling wild animals.

Surveillance efforts were also strengthened to track the occurrence of outbreaks and identify new cases. The focus was on establishing effective surveillance systems in areas known to be endemic for monkeypox, allowing for timely detection and response to outbreaks.

Infection control measures were also implemented, particularly in healthcare settings. These measures emphasized the importance of isolation for infected individuals, the use of personal protective equipment (PPE) by healthcare workers, and the proper disinfection of contaminated materials.

While these efforts were largely successful in containing outbreaks, the limited resources available in many African countries presented a significant challenge. The lack of adequate infrastructure, healthcare facilities, and trained personnel often hampered public health efforts and hindered the effectiveness of interventions.

2.5 Expanding Horizons: The First Cases Outside Africa

While monkeypox outbreaks remained primarily confined to Central and West Africa during the 1980s and 1990s, the virus was also detected in a few isolated cases outside the endemic region. These cases, though rare, served as a stark reminder of the virus's potential for global spread.

In 1986, a case of monkeypox was reported in the United States, in a laboratory worker who had been exposed to the virus during research activities. The case, though isolated, highlighted the potential for the virus to spread through laboratory settings and prompted a review of safety protocols for handling and studying monkeypox.

The 1990s saw a few more isolated cases of monkeypox reported outside Africa, including cases in the United Kingdom, Israel, and Singapore. These cases were linked to travel from endemic regions, suggesting the potential for the virus to be introduced to non-endemic areas through international travel and trade.

These isolated cases, though seemingly insignificant, served as early warning signs, suggesting the potential for monkeypox to emerge as a global health threat. They highlighted the need for increased vigilance, improved surveillance, and a coordinated international response to prevent the spread of the virus beyond its endemic region.

2.6 A Growing Concern: The Potential for a Pandemic

The emergence of monkeypox outbreaks in the 1980s and 1990s, along with the isolated cases reported outside Africa, raised a growing concern about the potential for the virus to become a global pandemic.

The increasing interconnectedness of the world, fueled by globalization, international travel, and trade, created new pathways for infectious diseases to spread. The potential for monkeypox to be introduced to non-endemic areas through travel, trade, or the movement of infected animals was a growing concern.

Furthermore, the lack of a specific treatment and the limited availability of vaccines for monkeypox added to the anxiety surrounding the potential for a pandemic. The global community recognized the need for proactive measures to prevent the spread of the virus and prepare for a potential outbreak.

The early outbreaks of monkeypox, though confined to Africa, served as a stark warning. They highlighted the potential for emerging infectious diseases to emerge from the depths of the natural world and disrupt the delicate balance of human health. The next decade would bring new challenges and a greater understanding of the virus's potential to spread and impact the global community.

2.7 The Legacy of the Early Outbreaks

The early outbreaks of monkeypox in the 1980s and 1990s, while limited in scope, were pivotal in shaping our understanding of the virus and its potential impact on human health. These outbreaks, coupled with the isolated cases reported outside Africa, served as a stark reminder of the importance of public health surveillance, early detection, and rapid response to emerging infectious diseases.

The early years of research into monkeypox also yielded valuable insights into the virus's transmission dynamics, its natural reservoir, and its potential for spread. The knowledge gained from these early outbreaks laid the groundwork for future research and public health interventions, ultimately paving the way for a more effective response to subsequent outbreaks.

The legacy of the early monkeypox outbreaks is a testament to the importance of global collaboration and the need for proactive measures to address emerging infectious diseases. The lessons learned from these early encounters with the virus would prove to be invaluable in preparing the world for the challenges that lay ahead.

As we move into the next chapter, we will explore the emergence of monkeypox in the United States, an event that marked a turning point in the global response to this emerging infectious disease.

Chapter 3: Emergence in the United States (2003)

3.1 A Shocking Awakening: Monkeypox Crosses the Atlantic

The year is 2003. The world, while grappling with the ongoing threat of SARS, a respiratory virus that emerged from China, was seemingly oblivious to a new threat brewing on the horizon. This threat, however, was not a new virus but one that had long lurked in the shadows of the African rainforest: monkeypox. The virus, which had been confined primarily to Central and West Africa for decades, was about to make a dramatic entrance onto the global stage, landing on American soil and shaking the nation's public health system to its core.

The first signs of the impending outbreak appeared in the spring of 2003, when a series of unusual cases emerged in the Midwest, specifically in Wisconsin and Illinois. The patients, initially misdiagnosed with chickenpox or smallpox, presented with the characteristic symptoms of monkeypox: fever, headache, muscle aches, and a distinctive rash that evolved into pustules.

The outbreak was unusual, not only for its location but also for the scale of the outbreak. Unlike previous outbreaks in Africa, which were typically limited in scope, this outbreak quickly expanded, impacting dozens of people. The puzzle began to unravel when the investigation revealed a common link between the patients: they had all come into contact with pet prairie dogs, a popular exotic pet in the United States.

The discovery of the prairie dog connection sent shockwaves through the scientific and public health communities. The prairie dog, a native North American species, had never been implicated in monkeypox transmission before. The emergence of this outbreak, involving a seemingly innocuous pet, highlighted the unpredictable nature of infectious diseases and the potential for their rapid spread through previously unknown pathways.

3.2 Tracing the Trail: Unveiling the Importation Route

The investigation into the 2003 monkeypox outbreak quickly turned into a global detective story, tracing the virus's journey from its African origin to the heartland of America. The trail led back to Ghana, a country in West Africa where the virus is endemic.

The investigation revealed that the prairie dogs, imported from Ghana as exotic pets, had been housed in a facility alongside other animals, including Gambian giant pouched rats, a known reservoir for monkeypox. The virus, likely transmitted from the rats to the prairie dogs, had then spread to humans through close contact with the infected pets.

The importation of infected prairie dogs into the United States was a significant turning point in the history of monkeypox. The outbreak, the first of its kind outside Africa, demonstrated the potential for global travel and trade to facilitate the spread of infectious diseases. It also highlighted the vulnerability of the global community to emerging pathogens, particularly those with zoonotic origins.

3.3 The Global Response: A Collaborative Effort

The emergence of monkeypox in the United States triggered a swift and coordinated response from the global public health community. The World Health Organization (WHO) and the Centers for Disease Control and Prevention (CDC) collaborated to investigate the outbreak, provide guidance on containment measures, and develop strategies to prevent future outbreaks.

The response involved a multi-faceted approach, including:

- **Surveillance and Contact Tracing:** Public health officials conducted rigorous surveillance to identify new cases and prevent further spread. Contact tracing was implemented to identify individuals who had been in contact with infected individuals or animals, allowing for early intervention and isolation.

- **Isolation and Quarantine:** Infected individuals were isolated to prevent further spread, while individuals who had been in close contact with infected individuals were quarantined to monitor for signs of infection.

- **Vaccination:** The availability of a smallpox vaccine, which offered cross-protection against monkeypox, played a crucial role in controlling the outbreak. However, the limited supply of the vaccine and the need to prioritize individuals at highest risk made it a challenge to vaccinate everyone who could have been exposed.

- **Animal Control and Quarantine:** The outbreak prompted a ban on the importation of prairie dogs from Ghana and other countries known to be endemic for monkeypox. Quarantine measures were also implemented for animals that had been in contact with infected individuals, to prevent further spread.

- **Public Education and Awareness:** Public health officials launched widespread public education campaigns to raise awareness about monkeypox, its symptoms, and preventive measures. The campaigns emphasized the importance of avoiding contact with exotic animals and the need for vigilance in case of potential exposure.

The global response to the 2003 monkeypox outbreak demonstrated the importance of international collaboration and rapid response in addressing emerging infectious diseases. The lessons learned from this outbreak would shape future public health efforts to prevent and control the spread of monkeypox and other emerging pathogens.

3.4 The Aftermath: A Turning Point in Public Health Preparedness

The 2003 monkeypox outbreak, while ultimately contained, left an indelible mark on the global public health landscape. The outbreak served as a stark reminder of the potential for emerging infectious diseases to pose a significant threat to public health, particularly in the era of globalization and increasing travel and trade.

The outbreak prompted a reassessment of public health preparedness strategies, emphasizing the need for robust surveillance systems, rapid response mechanisms, and a coordinated global effort to address emerging threats.

The outbreak also highlighted the importance of understanding the role of wildlife in infectious disease transmission and the need to address the growing issue of zoonotic diseases.

The 2003 monkeypox outbreak was a watershed moment in the global fight against infectious diseases. It served as a catalyst for increased research, surveillance, and public health preparedness efforts. The lessons learned from this outbreak would prove to be invaluable in the years to come, as the world grappled with new and emerging threats to human health.

3.5 The Lasting Impact: A Legacy of Vigilance

The 2003 monkeypox outbreak, while relatively small compared to subsequent outbreaks, had a profound impact on public health preparedness in the United States and globally. It highlighted the importance of several key factors:

1. Surveillance and Early Detection: The outbreak underscored the need for robust surveillance systems, capable of detecting emerging infectious diseases at the earliest stages. Early detection is crucial for rapid containment and prevention of widespread outbreaks.

2. Rapid Response Mechanisms: The outbreak highlighted the need for well-coordinated, multi-agency response teams, capable of responding quickly and effectively to outbreaks. Effective response mechanisms involve collaboration among public health officials, healthcare providers, and other stakeholders.

3. International Collaboration: The global nature of the outbreak underscored the importance of international collaboration in addressing emerging infectious diseases. This includes sharing information, resources, and expertise to effectively prevent and control outbreaks across borders.

4. Zoonotic Disease Awareness: The outbreak highlighted the importance of understanding the role of wildlife in infectious disease transmission. Public health efforts should include measures to prevent the emergence of zoonotic diseases, such as strengthening animal health surveillance and promoting safe handling practices for animals.

5. Public Education and Engagement: The outbreak highlighted the importance of public education and engagement in preventing and controlling the spread of infectious diseases. Public awareness campaigns can educate individuals about the risks, symptoms, and prevention measures, empowering them to protect themselves and their communities.

The lessons learned from the 2003 monkeypox outbreak continue to shape public health policy and practices around the world. The outbreak served as a wake-up call, prompting a renewed focus on preparedness for emerging infectious diseases. The world, once seemingly oblivious to the threat posed by monkeypox, had been given a stark reminder of the potential for this virus to emerge as a global health threat.

3.6 A Look Ahead: New Challenges and Emerging Threats

While the 2003 monkeypox outbreak was a significant event in the history of the virus, it was only the beginning of a story that would unfold in the years to come. The decades following the 2003 outbreak witnessed a surge in monkeypox activity, particularly in Africa, where the virus remained endemic.

The emergence of monkeypox in the United States, however, had a lasting impact on global public health preparedness. It highlighted the importance of understanding the role of wildlife in infectious disease transmission, the potential for global travel and trade to facilitate the spread of pathogens, and the need for robust surveillance and response mechanisms to address emerging threats.

The world, now more aware of the potential for monkeypox to spread beyond its traditional endemic region, was better prepared for future outbreaks. The lessons learned from the 2003 outbreak would prove invaluable in navigating the challenges of the 2020s, when monkeypox would once again emerge as a global health threat.

The next chapter explores the continued activity of monkeypox in Africa in the 2000s and 2010s, a period that witnessed a surge in outbreaks, highlighting the persistent threat posed by this virus.

Chapter 4: Continued Activity in Africa (2000s-2010s)

4.1 A Persistent Threat: Monkeypox Endures in its Endemic Region

The 2000s and 2010s marked a period of continued monkeypox activity in its endemic region, primarily Central and West Africa. While the 2003 outbreak in the United States had served as a global wake-up call, highlighting the virus's potential for international spread, monkeypox remained a persistent threat in its traditional home, a silent, recurring burden on communities accustomed to its presence.

Despite the limited resources available in many African countries, public health authorities and researchers diligently tracked the virus's activity, documenting the patterns of outbreaks, gathering epidemiological data, and refining their understanding of the virus's complex transmission dynamics. These efforts, though hampered by logistical challenges and limited funding, yielded crucial insights into the virus's behavior and provided valuable data for developing more effective prevention and control strategies.

4.2 The Patterns of Outbreaks: Regional Variations and Seasonal Trends

During the 2000s and 2010s, monkeypox outbreaks continued to occur in Central and West Africa, primarily concentrated in countries like the Democratic Republic of Congo (DRC), Nigeria, Cameroon, Gabon, and Sierra Leone. These outbreaks were often sporadic, with periods of relative inactivity followed by sudden surges in cases.

The outbreaks often displayed distinct regional variations, reflecting the unique ecological and social factors in each region. For example, in the DRC, a country with a vast and diverse landscape, outbreaks were frequently reported in rural areas, often associated with contact with infected rodents. In Nigeria, a country with a high population density, outbreaks were more likely to occur in urban areas, driven by human-to-human transmission.

The timing of outbreaks also exhibited seasonal trends, often coinciding with periods of increased contact with infected animals, such as during the harvest season or during periods of heavy rainfall when rodents were more active. This seasonal pattern, though not consistently observed across all regions, highlighted the importance of environmental factors in driving the virus's spread.

4.3 Understanding the Transmission Dynamics: The Complex Interplay of Host Factors

The outbreaks in the 2000s and 2010s provided valuable insights into the transmission dynamics of monkeypox, revealing the complex interplay of host factors that contribute to the virus's spread. The primary mode of transmission remained direct contact with infected animals, particularly rodents, through bites, scratches, or handling contaminated carcasses. However, human-to-human transmission, through close contact with infected individuals, particularly through respiratory droplets or direct contact with infected lesions, became increasingly recognized as a significant factor.

Research revealed that monkeypox could be transmitted through various routes:

- **Direct Contact with Infected Animals:** This remained the most common mode of transmission, particularly in rural communities where close contact with rodents was frequent. Hunting, farming, and other activities involving the handling of wild animals posed a significant risk.

- **Human-to-Human Transmission:** This mode of transmission became increasingly recognized, particularly in urban settings where close contact between infected individuals was more likely. Transmission could occur through respiratory droplets, direct contact with infected lesions, or through contaminated materials.

- **Indirect Contact:** The virus could also be spread through indirect contact with contaminated materials, such as bedding, clothing, or other objects that had been in contact with infected individuals or animals.

The emergence of human-to-human transmission, particularly in urban settings, highlighted the importance of public health interventions, such as isolation of infected individuals, contact tracing, and education campaigns, in preventing the spread of the virus.

4.4 The Role of Wildlife in the Transmission Cycle: Expanding the Reservoir

While rodents continued to be recognized as the primary reservoir of monkeypox, research in the 2000s and 2010s expanded our understanding of the virus's transmission cycle, highlighting the potential role of other wildlife species in the spread of the virus.

Studies revealed that various primate species, including monkeys, could become infected with monkeypox, particularly those that were kept as pets or were in close contact with humans. These primates, though not the primary reservoir, could serve as intermediate hosts, facilitating the transmission of the virus to humans.

The expanding list of potential hosts underscored the complexity of the monkeypox transmission cycle, highlighting the importance of understanding the virus's interactions with different animal species and the potential for spillover events from wildlife to humans.

4.5 The Impact of Outbreaks: Human Health Consequences and Socioeconomic Disruptions

Monkeypox outbreaks in Africa often had significant impacts on affected communities, both in terms of human health consequences and socioeconomic disruptions. The disease, while generally mild, could cause significant discomfort and, in rare cases, lead to complications like pneumonia, encephalitis, and even death.

The outbreaks could also disrupt daily life, causing fear, isolation, and stigma for infected individuals and their families. School closures, travel restrictions, and economic losses were often associated with outbreaks, particularly in remote areas where economies were heavily reliant on agriculture and trade.

The impact of monkeypox outbreaks highlighted the importance of public health interventions, such as prompt diagnosis, treatment, and isolation, in minimizing the human health consequences and socioeconomic disruptions associated with the disease.

4.6 The Challenges of Disease Management: Limited Resources and Infrastructure

Managing monkeypox outbreaks in Africa was often challenging, primarily due to limited resources and infrastructure in many endemic countries. The lack of adequate healthcare facilities, trained personnel, and diagnostic tools often hampered public health efforts and hindered the effectiveness of interventions.

The limited availability of antiviral treatments, such as cidofovir, which had shown some effectiveness in treating monkeypox, was a significant challenge. The cost of these treatments, along with the logistical difficulties of accessing them in remote areas, limited their use in many outbreaks.

Furthermore, the lack of a readily available vaccine, particularly for widespread use, remained a major obstacle in controlling the spread of the virus. While the smallpox vaccine offered cross-protection against monkeypox, its limited availability and the need to prioritize individuals at highest risk made it a challenge to implement vaccination programs effectively.

4.7 The Evolution of Public Health Responses: Strengthening Surveillance and Improving Interventions

The challenges of managing monkeypox outbreaks in Africa prompted a constant evolution of public health responses, focusing on strengthening surveillance systems, improving interventions, and enhancing collaboration among stakeholders.

- **Surveillance Systems:** Public health authorities in endemic countries worked diligently to improve surveillance systems, aiming to detect outbreaks early and track their spread more effectively. This involved establishing robust reporting systems, training personnel, and strengthening laboratory capacity for diagnosing the virus.

- **Interventions:** Efforts were made to improve interventions, particularly in terms of infection control measures, isolation of infected individuals, contact tracing, and public education campaigns. The focus was on promoting safe handling practices for animals, particularly rodents, and educating communities about the risks of the virus and how to prevent its spread.

- **Collaboration:** Collaboration among public health agencies, research institutions, and international organizations became increasingly critical in managing monkeypox outbreaks. This collaboration involved sharing information, resources, and expertise, working together to develop and implement more effective prevention and control strategies.

4.8 The Rise of Research and Development: Seeking New Tools to Combat the Virus

The continued activity of monkeypox in Africa prompted a renewed focus on research and development efforts to combat the virus, seeking to develop more effective diagnostic tools, antiviral treatments, and vaccines.

- **Diagnostic Tools:** Efforts were made to develop more readily available and accurate diagnostic tests, particularly for use in resource-limited settings. This involved exploring new technologies, such as polymerase chain reaction (PCR) tests, which could provide rapid and reliable diagnosis.

- **Antiviral Treatments:** Research into antiviral treatments continued, focusing on identifying existing medications that could be effective against monkeypox and exploring the development of new drugs.

- **Vaccines:** Research efforts aimed to develop new vaccines specifically for monkeypox, exploring different vaccine platforms and strategies to improve efficacy and safety.

The ongoing research efforts in the 2000s and 2010s reflected the growing concern about the potential for monkeypox to emerge as a global health threat, prompting a renewed focus on developing effective tools to prevent and control the virus.

4.9 A Shifting Paradigm: From Local Concern to Global Threat

While monkeypox remained a persistent threat in Africa, the outbreaks in the 2000s and 2010s were not confined to the continent. The virus was detected in isolated cases outside Africa, linked to travel from endemic regions. This sporadic spread, though limited in scope, highlighted the potential for the virus to emerge as a global threat.

The isolated cases, coupled with the ongoing research efforts to understand the virus's transmission dynamics and its potential for adaptation, signaled a shifting paradigm. Monkeypox, once considered a localized concern confined to Africa, was increasingly recognized as a potential global health threat.

4.10 The Legacy of Continued Activity in Africa: A Call to Action

The continued activity of monkeypox in Africa during the 2000s and 2010s, despite the global community's growing awareness of the virus's potential, served as a sobering reminder of the challenges posed by neglected tropical diseases.

These outbreaks underscored the need for sustained efforts to control the virus in its endemic region, focusing on improving surveillance, enhancing interventions, and supporting research and development for more effective tools.

The lessons learned from the outbreaks in Africa, particularly the importance of international collaboration, public health preparedness, and the role of wildlife in disease transmission, would prove to be invaluable in navigating the global challenges posed by monkeypox in the years to come.

4.11 Looking Ahead: The Emerging Global Threat

The 2010s witnessed a growing concern about the potential for monkeypox to emerge as a global health threat. The virus had already been detected in several countries outside Africa, linked to travel from endemic regions. The emergence of monkeypox in the United States in 2003 had served as a stark warning, highlighting the potential for the virus to be imported and spread through international travel and trade.

As the world became increasingly interconnected, the risk of monkeypox spreading globally was a growing concern. The virus's ability to spread through human-to-human transmission, particularly in densely populated urban areas, posed a new challenge.

The next chapter explores the emergence of monkeypox as a global concern in the 2020s, a period marked by a rapid surge in cases and a renewed focus on global health preparedness.

Chapter 5: Global Concern and Spread (2020s)

5.1 Monkeypox Takes Center Stage

The year is 2022. The world, still reeling from the COVID-19 pandemic, finds itself confronting a new, emerging threat: a resurgence of monkeypox. This time, however, the virus is no longer confined to its traditional endemic regions in Central and West Africa. Monkeypox, once a relatively obscure disease, has unexpectedly taken center stage, spreading rapidly across continents and igniting a global health crisis.

The emergence of monkeypox as a global concern in the 2020s marks a significant shift in the virus's history. The virus, which had been circulating in Africa for decades, had shown sporadic evidence of spreading beyond the continent, but the outbreaks remained isolated and relatively contained. However, the events of 2022 and beyond revealed a new and unsettling reality: monkeypox had become a global pandemic, a threat capable of impacting populations worldwide.

5.2 The Surge in Cases: A Global Outbreak Unfolds

The first signs of the global monkeypox outbreak emerged in early 2022, when a series of cases were reported in Europe, primarily in the United Kingdom and Portugal. These cases were initially linked to travel from West African countries, particularly Nigeria, where monkeypox was endemic. However, as the number of cases grew, it became clear that the outbreak was not simply a result of imported cases but was spreading through human-to-human transmission.

The outbreak quickly expanded, spreading to countries across Europe, North America, South America, Asia, and Australia. By the end of 2022, the World Health Organization (WHO) had reported over 80,000 cases in over 100 countries, a significant increase from the few hundred cases reported annually in previous years.

The rapid spread of monkeypox across continents was a concerning development, raising questions about the virus's ability to adapt to new environments and its potential for sustained transmission in non-endemic regions. The outbreak also highlighted the vulnerability of the global community to emerging infectious diseases, particularly those with zoonotic origins.

5.3 A New Transmission Pattern: Human-to-Human Transmission Takes Center Stage

One of the most striking features of the global monkeypox outbreak was the dominance of human-to-human transmission. Unlike previous outbreaks, which were primarily linked to contact with infected animals, the 2022 outbreak primarily involved transmission between humans through close contact, particularly skin-to-skin contact with infected lesions or respiratory droplets.

The shift to human-to-human transmission was likely due to several factors, including:

- **Increased International Travel and Trade:** The global nature of the outbreak was likely fueled by increased international travel and trade, which facilitated the movement of infected individuals across borders.

- **Changes in Social Behavior:** The outbreak coincided with a period of increased social activity and close contact between individuals, following the easing of COVID-19 restrictions.

- **Changes in Sexual Behavior:** The outbreak was disproportionately impacting individuals who identified as men who have sex with men (MSM), suggesting that close physical contact during sexual activity may play a significant role in transmission.

- **Increased Awareness:** The global outbreak led to increased awareness of monkeypox and its symptoms, leading to more individuals seeking testing and diagnosis.

The dominance of human-to-human transmission presented a new challenge in controlling the outbreak, as it increased the potential for sustained transmission in non-endemic regions. Public health officials faced the task of rapidly scaling up testing and contact tracing efforts to identify and isolate infected individuals, prevent further spread.

5.4 Unraveling the Outbreak: The Role of Animal Reservoirs

While human-to-human transmission was the primary driver of the global monkeypox outbreak, the virus's origins remained linked to its natural reservoir in animals. While the exact source of the 2022 outbreak was not definitively identified, investigations pointed to several potential animal reservoirs:

- **Rodents:** Rodents, particularly the African giant pouched rat (Cricetomys gambianus), were considered the primary reservoir of monkeypox. The virus was known to circulate among rodents in West Africa, and there was evidence that the virus could be transmitted from rodents to humans through bites, scratches, or contact with contaminated carcasses.

- **Primates:** Several primate species, including monkeys, were also known to be susceptible to monkeypox infection. There was evidence that primates could serve as intermediate hosts, facilitating the transmission of the virus from rodents to humans.

- **Other Wildlife Species:** The potential role of other wildlife species in the transmission cycle, particularly those that come into contact with humans, remained an active area of investigation.

The investigation into the animal reservoirs of monkeypox was crucial for understanding the virus's origins and for developing effective strategies to prevent future outbreaks. Efforts were made to strengthen surveillance of wildlife populations in endemic regions and to promote safe handling practices for animals.

5.5 A Race Against Time: Global Response and Control Measures

The global monkeypox outbreak triggered a coordinated response from the international community, with public health agencies, research institutions, and international organizations working together to contain the spread of the virus. The response involved a multi-faceted approach, including:

- **Surveillance and Contact Tracing:** Public health officials implemented rigorous surveillance measures to identify new cases and track the spread of the virus. Contact tracing was used to identify individuals who had been in close contact with infected individuals, allowing for early intervention and isolation.

- **Isolation and Quarantine:** Infected individuals were isolated to prevent further spread, while individuals who had been in close contact with infected individuals were quarantined to monitor for signs of infection.

- **Vaccination:** The availability of a smallpox vaccine, which offered cross-protection against monkeypox, played a crucial role in controlling the outbreak. However, the limited supply of the vaccine and the need to prioritize individuals at highest risk made it a challenge to vaccinate everyone who could have been exposed.

- **Antiviral Treatments:** Antiviral medications, such as tecovirimat (TPOXX) and brincidofovir (CMX001), were available for treating monkeypox, but they were not readily available in all countries, and their use was often limited to severe cases.

- **Public Education and Awareness:** Public health officials launched widespread public education campaigns to raise awareness about monkeypox, its symptoms, and preventive measures. The campaigns emphasized the importance of avoiding close contact with infected individuals, practicing good hygiene, and seeking medical attention if they developed any symptoms.

- **Research and Development:** The outbreak prompted renewed efforts to develop more effective diagnostic tools, antiviral treatments, and vaccines specifically for monkeypox. Research was also ongoing to improve our understanding of the virus's transmission dynamics and its potential for adaptation.

5.6 Navigating Challenges: Inequalities in Access to Treatment and Vaccines

The global monkeypox outbreak highlighted the stark inequalities in access to healthcare and resources around the world. The availability of vaccines and antiviral treatments varied significantly across countries, with limited access in many low- and middle-income countries.

This inequity in access to resources posed a significant challenge in controlling the outbreak, as it allowed the virus to continue spreading in regions with limited access to prevention and treatment measures.

The situation highlighted the need for a more equitable distribution of vaccines, treatments, and diagnostic tools, particularly in countries most vulnerable to emerging infectious diseases. The global community faced the challenge of ensuring that everyone had equal access to the resources needed to prevent and control outbreaks.

5.7 The Impact on Individuals and Communities

The global monkeypox outbreak had a significant impact on individuals and communities worldwide. The disease, while generally mild, could cause significant discomfort and, in rare cases, lead to complications. The outbreak also resulted in social stigma and discrimination, particularly for individuals who identified as MSM, who were disproportionately affected by the outbreak.

The outbreak had a profound impact on mental health, with many individuals experiencing anxiety, fear, and social isolation. The outbreak also disrupted daily life, causing school closures, travel restrictions, and economic losses.

5.8 Lessons Learned: Building a More Resilient Global Health System

The global monkeypox outbreak, while challenging, provided valuable lessons for building a more resilient global health system. The outbreak highlighted the need for:

- **Enhanced Surveillance Systems:** Robust surveillance systems, capable of detecting emerging infectious diseases early and tracking their spread, are crucial for preventing and controlling outbreaks.

- **Rapid Response Mechanisms:** Well-coordinated, multi-agency response teams, capable of responding quickly and effectively to outbreaks, are essential for containing the spread of emerging pathogens.

- **Global Collaboration:** International collaboration, including the sharing of information, resources, and expertise, is critical for addressing global health threats.

- **Equitable Access to Resources:** Ensuring equitable access to vaccines, treatments, and diagnostic tools is crucial for protecting all populations, particularly those most vulnerable to emerging infectious diseases.

- **Preparedness for Zoonotic Diseases:** Understanding the role of wildlife in disease transmission and strengthening surveillance of animal populations is essential for preventing future outbreaks.

5.9 A New Era of Vigilance: The Challenges Ahead

The global monkeypox outbreak of 2022 and beyond marked a turning point in the history of this virus. The outbreak demonstrated the virus's potential to emerge as a global health threat, highlighting the need for sustained vigilance and preparedness.

The challenges ahead include:

- **Controlling the Spread:** The ongoing challenge of controlling the spread of the virus, particularly through human-to-human transmission, remains a priority.

- **Developing Effective Vaccines and Treatments:** Efforts to develop more effective vaccines and treatments for monkeypox, particularly those that are readily available and affordable, are crucial.

- **Addressing Inequalities in Access to Healthcare:** The global community must work towards addressing the inequalities in access to healthcare resources, ensuring that everyone has equal access to the tools needed to prevent and control infectious diseases.

- **Preparedness for Future Outbreaks:** The global community must learn from the experiences of the monkeypox outbreak, strengthening surveillance systems, improving response mechanisms, and investing in research and development to prepare for future emerging infectious diseases.

5.10 The Road Ahead: A Call to Action

The global monkeypox outbreak, while a significant health crisis, has also presented a valuable opportunity to strengthen the global health system. The lessons learned from the outbreak can inform a more proactive and collaborative approach to preventing and controlling emerging infectious diseases.

The road ahead requires a collective effort, with nations, organizations, and individuals working together to:

- **Invest in Public Health:** Increase investments in public health infrastructure, surveillance systems, and research and development, to enhance preparedness for future outbreaks.

- **Strengthen International Collaboration:** Promote global collaboration and data sharing to effectively track and respond to emerging infectious diseases.

- **Address Health Inequalities:** Work towards reducing health disparities and ensuring equitable access to healthcare resources, particularly in low- and middle-income countries.

- **Increase Public Awareness:** Promote public awareness about emerging infectious diseases and the importance of preventive measures.

The global monkeypox outbreak has served as a stark reminder of the interconnectedness of our world and the potential for infectious diseases to cross borders and impact populations worldwide. The lessons learned from this outbreak can guide us toward a more resilient and equitable global health system, one that is better prepared to face the challenges of emerging infectious diseases.

Chapter 6: Ongoing Developments (2023-Present)

6.1 The Shifting Tide: A Global Response Evolves

The global monkeypox outbreak, which exploded onto the world stage in 2022, continued to dominate public health discussions and research efforts throughout 2023 and beyond. While the initial surge of cases subsided, the virus remained a persistent threat, particularly in certain regions, and its long-term implications for global health remained a significant area of concern.

The response to the outbreak, which initially focused on containment and mitigation, gradually shifted towards a more sustainable approach, emphasizing long-term preparedness, vaccine development, and a deeper understanding of the virus's dynamics. The lessons learned from the initial phase of the outbreak informed a more nuanced and collaborative approach to managing the virus's ongoing presence.

The global monkeypox outbreak of 2022 and beyond can be viewed as two distinct phases:

Phase 1: The Initial Surge (2022)

This phase was characterized by a rapid increase in cases, primarily driven by human-to-human transmission, particularly through close physical contact. The outbreak spread rapidly across continents, prompting a global response focused on containment, isolation, and vaccination. The initial surge highlighted the virus's capacity for rapid spread in non-endemic regions and the challenges of responding to a novel outbreak in a highly interconnected world.

Phase 2: The Shift to Endemic Transmission (2023 - Present)

As the initial surge subsided, the monkeypox outbreak transitioned into a more complex and persistent stage. The virus continued to circulate in certain regions, particularly in West and Central Africa, where it had long been endemic. In these regions, the virus continued to cause sporadic outbreaks, primarily linked to contact with infected animals.

Outside of these endemic regions, the outbreak transitioned into a pattern of sporadic cases, often linked to travel from endemic areas or to ongoing transmission within smaller, interconnected communities. This second phase highlighted the challenge of managing a virus that had established a foothold in new environments and the importance of ongoing surveillance and targeted interventions.

6.3 The Global Response Evolves: A Focus on Preparedness and Sustainability

The response to the monkeypox outbreak shifted significantly from the initial emergency phase to a more long-term, sustainable approach, driven by the following key elements:

1. Strengthening Surveillance Systems: Global health agencies and national public health organizations worked to improve surveillance systems, aiming to detect new cases early and track the virus's spread more effectively. This involved expanding testing capacity, improving data collection and analysis, and strengthening laboratory networks.

2. Developing More Effective Vaccines: The global response prioritized the development of new vaccines specifically for monkeypox. The existing smallpox vaccine, which offered cross-protection against monkeypox, remained a crucial tool, but its limited availability and the potential for side effects spurred the development of more targeted and effective vaccines.

3. Expanding Access to Treatment: Efforts focused on ensuring wider access to antiviral treatments for monkeypox, particularly in low- and middle-income countries. The cost and availability of these treatments remained a significant barrier, prompting initiatives to increase affordability and improve distribution networks.

4. Addressing Health Disparities: The response acknowledged the disproportionate impact of monkeypox on certain communities, particularly individuals who identified as MSM, and emphasized the need for targeted interventions and outreach programs to address these disparities.

5. Promoting Public Health Education: Public health campaigns aimed to raise awareness about monkeypox, its symptoms, and preventive measures, particularly in communities at higher risk of exposure.

6. Improving International Collaboration: The global response highlighted the need for stronger international collaboration in tracking the virus, sharing resources, and coordinating research efforts. The World Health Organization played a crucial role in coordinating the response, providing guidance, and supporting countries with limited resources.

6.4 A Surge in Research: Unveiling the Virus's Secrets

The global monkeypox outbreak reignited research efforts into the virus, prompting a surge in studies focused on understanding its transmission dynamics, its potential for adaptation, and the development of new vaccines and treatments.

1. Understanding Transmission Dynamics: Researchers conducted studies to better understand how the virus spreads, exploring the role of different modes of transmission, including respiratory droplets, skin-to-skin contact, and contaminated materials. The goal was to identify key factors contributing to the spread of the virus and to develop more effective infection control measures.

2. Investigating Potential Reservoirs: The search for the animal reservoirs of monkeypox continued, with researchers investigating potential roles for various rodent species, primates, and other wildlife species. The goal was to identify the source of the virus and to develop strategies to prevent future spillover events from animals to humans.

3. Studying Viral Evolution: Researchers analyzed the virus's genetic makeup, tracking its evolution and identifying potential mutations that could impact its transmissibility or its response to vaccines and treatments. This research provided valuable insights into the virus's adaptation and its potential for developing resistance to interventions.

4. Developing New Vaccines: Research efforts focused on developing new vaccines specifically for monkeypox, exploring different vaccine platforms and strategies to improve efficacy, safety, and ease of administration. The goal was to develop vaccines that could be more readily available, more effective, and more widely accessible, particularly in resource-limited settings.

5. Searching for Effective Treatments: The search for new and effective antiviral treatments for monkeypox continued, exploring existing medications that could be repurposed and developing new drugs with potential efficacy against the virus. The goal was to identify treatments that were safe, effective, and readily available, particularly for individuals with severe cases of the disease.

6.5 The Global Impact: A Ripple Effect

The global monkeypox outbreak had a profound impact on the global health landscape, extending beyond the immediate health consequences. The outbreak served as a stark reminder of the interconnectedness of our world and the vulnerability of global health to emerging infectious diseases.

1. Strengthening Global Health Preparedness: The outbreak prompted a renewed focus on global health preparedness, with countries and organizations investing in strengthening surveillance systems, improving response mechanisms, and building a more resilient global health infrastructure.

2. Addressing Health Disparities: The outbreak highlighted the significant health disparities that exist around the world, particularly in access to healthcare and resources. This prompted calls for a more equitable distribution of vaccines, treatments, and diagnostic tools, ensuring that everyone has equal access to the resources needed to prevent and control infectious diseases.

3. Promoting One Health: The outbreak emphasized the importance of a One Health approach to infectious diseases, recognizing the interconnectedness of human health, animal health, and environmental health. This approach emphasized the need for collaboration across disciplines and sectors to prevent and control diseases that emerge from animal reservoirs.

4. Improving Communication and Transparency: The outbreak underscored the importance of clear, accurate, and timely communication about infectious diseases. Effective communication can help to dispel myths, reduce fear, and promote public understanding and cooperation in controlling outbreaks.

6.6 A Call to Action: Building a More Resilient Future

The ongoing monkeypox outbreak, while a significant challenge, has presented a valuable opportunity to strengthen the global health system and to build a more resilient future. This requires a collective effort from governments, organizations, and individuals to address the following key priorities:

- **Invest in Public Health:** Increase investments in public health infrastructure, surveillance systems, research and development, and training to improve preparedness for future outbreaks.

- **Strengthen International Collaboration:** Foster strong partnerships between countries and organizations to share information, resources, and expertise, ensuring a coordinated global response to emerging infectious diseases.

- **Address Health Disparities:** Work towards reducing health disparities and ensuring equitable access to healthcare resources, particularly in low- and middle-income countries.

- **Promote One Health:** Encourage a One Health approach to infectious diseases, emphasizing the interconnectedness of human health, animal health, and environmental health.

- **Improve Communication and Transparency:** Prioritize clear, accurate, and timely communication about infectious diseases to build public trust and promote informed decision-making.

The global monkeypox outbreak has served as a stark reminder of the fragility of global health and the need for collective action to prevent and control emerging infectious diseases. By learning from the experiences of this outbreak, we can build a more resilient and equitable global health system, one that is better equipped to face the challenges of the future.

6.7 The Uncertain Future: The Legacy of Monkeypox

The legacy of the monkeypox outbreak remains to be written, its full implications unfolding in the years to come. The virus, once a relatively obscure threat confined to Africa, has emerged as a global concern, reminding us of the constant threat posed by emerging infectious diseases.

The outbreak has prompted a significant shift in our understanding of the virus, its transmission dynamics, and its potential for global spread. It has also highlighted the need for a more proactive and collaborative approach to global health, emphasizing the importance of preparedness, surveillance, and equity.

While the initial surge of cases subsided, the virus continues to circulate in certain regions, and its long-term impact on global health remains to be seen. The ongoing research efforts, the development of new vaccines and treatments, and the lessons learned from the outbreak will continue to shape our response to this virus and to other emerging infectious diseases.

The future of monkeypox, like the future of global health, is uncertain. However, the lessons learned from this outbreak can serve as a guide, prompting us to work together to build a more resilient and equitable world, one that is better prepared to face the challenges of emerging infectious diseases and to protect the health of all people.

9 798336 885507